Marburg:

I0410140

The Deadly Virus That Threatens Us All

Kelli Boone

Table of contents

CHAPTER 4: THE FUTURE OF MARBURG VIRUS DISEASE

What are the challenges of preventing and treating MVD?

What are the prospects for a vaccine?

CHAPTER 5: MARBURG VIRUS DISEASE: WHAT YOU CAN DO

What can communities and governments do to prevent

and respond to MVD outbreaks?

Conclusion

INTRODUCTION

The Marburg virus, a lethal pathogen that belongs to the family Filoviridae, has drawn attention from all around the world due to its propensity to lead to major epidemics of hemorrhagic fever. It has many destructive traits with the more well-known Ebola virus and was named after the German city of Marburg, where the virus was initially discovered in 1967.

The Marburg virus is categorized as a pathogen with a biosafety level of 4 (BSL-4), which is indicative of the strict containment procedures necessary to study and handle it. It is the cause of Marburg virus disease (MVD), a rare but serious condition that can have a high fatality rate in those who contract it. Fever, chills, malaise, and, in more severe cases, bleeding issues and organ failure are some of the symptoms of MVD.

In the past, Marburg virus outbreaks have been rare and frequently linked to close contact between people and afflicted animals like bats and primates. Direct contact with the blood, saliva, organs, or other bodily fluids of infected people can also result in human-to-human transmission. Marburg virus is a significant public health concern due to its propensity for fast and sustained transmission across healthcare environments and communities.

In order to set the stage for a more in-depth investigation of the characteristics, transmission, clinical symptoms, preventive, and control strategies of the Marburg virus, this introduction seeks to provide a succinct summary of the disease. In order to reduce the effects of possible outbreaks and create efficient treatments and vaccinations, it is imperative for public health efforts to comprehend the nature of this virus.

CHAPTER 1: MARBURG VIRUS DISEASE: WHAT YOU NEED TO KNOW

The Marburg virus is the cause of Marburg Virus Disease, also known as MVD, a serious and extremely contagious sickness. Understanding the fundamentals of this illness is crucial because this lethal bacteria poses a serious threat to the general public's health.

Origin and Discovery

When the Marburg virus outbreak broke out in the German city of Marburg in 1967, researchers realized that the illness had its roots in Africa. Accidental laboratory worker exposure to the tissues and blood samples of imported African green monkeys used for research was the cause of this outbreak. These workers developed a mystery, severe sickness with multiple organ failure, a high fever, and bleeding tendencies.

Medical authorities quickly responded to segregate and treat the affected people after realizing how terrible the situation was. The novel virus that caused the outbreak was found after blood and tissue samples from the affected patients were sent to labs for analysis. This signaled the emergence of the filoviridae family's new, distinct, and dangerous pathogen, the Marburg virus illness, which is closely related to the Ebola virus.

Since its initial discovery, the Marburg virus disease has intermittently appeared in a number of African countries, frequently linked to activities that put people in close proximity to afflicted wildlife, especially bats and primates. Understanding and controlling this fatal disease still rely heavily on continuing research into its causes and transmission patterns.

How is MVD transmitted?

The main way that the Marburg virus disease (MVD) is spread is through direct contact with an infected person's bodily fluids. When someone comes into touch with blood, saliva, vomit, urine, feces, or other fluids from an infected person, the virus is disseminated.

The danger of transmission is greatly increased by close personal contact, such as tending to or touching an infected person without taking the proper precautions. Additionally, because the virus can survive in dead corpses for some time after death, MVD can be acquired via handling the remains of people who have died with the illness.

Healthcare facilities present a special danger for virus transmission due to contaminated medical equipment and insufficient infection control procedures. Healthcare professionals in these settings are at a greater risk of developing MVD when caring for infected patients without the appropriate protective equipment.

MVD epidemics have occasionally been connected to consuming infected wildlife, especially bats and non-human primates. Without taking the necessary precautions, those who handle, butcher, or consume these animals run the danger of getting sick.

For the purpose of establishing efficient preventative measures and containing the spread of this incredibly contagious and fatal disease, it is essential to understand the Marburg virus's routes of transmission.

What are the symptoms of MVD?

The Marburg virus disease (MVD) symptoms appear suddenly and severely, and they consist of the following:

1. High fever: MVD frequently starts with a fever that exceeds 101°F (38.3°C). One of the first and most noticeable signs is this fever.

2. Chills: As the fever increases, patients shiver violently and have the chills.

3. Weakness and weariness: Patients frequently experience profound weakness and acute weariness, as well as feeling lethargic and depleted of energy.

4. Headache: A common symptom of MVD is severe headaches that are frequently described as throbbing or pounding.

5. Severe joint and muscle pain: Patients may endure excruciating joint and muscle pain, which can be incapacitating.

6. Nausea and Vomiting: These gastrointestinal symptoms of MVD are frequent and might cause dehydration.

7. Abdominal Pain: Patients may have discomfort and pain in their abdomen, which is frequently accompanied by diarrhea.

8. Chest Pain and Cough: People with MVD sometimes feel chest pain and a chronic cough.

9. Hemorrhagic Symptoms: Severe MVD patients may experience bleeding tendencies, which can cause symptoms like easy bruising, bloody vomit, bloody diarrhea, bleeding gums, and nasal bleeding.

10. Organ Failure: As the illness worsens, numerous organ systems may be impacted, which can cause respiratory distress, cardiovascular collapse, liver and kidney failure, and other symptoms like liver and kidney dysfunction.

Rapid MVD progression can cause severe cases to quickly pass away, sometimes from multiple organ failure and shock. For the best chance of survival, especially in areas where the Marburg virus is endemic or when outbreaks are present, it is imperative to identify these symptoms early and seek rapid medical assistance.

How is MVD diagnosed?

MVD diagnosis comprises a number of essential processes and diagnostic procedures, including:

1. Clinical Assessment: Physicians begin by evaluating the patient's clinical presentation, noting symptoms including fever, muscle

discomfort, and weakness as well as any possible history of virus exposure, such as recent travel to an area where the virus is endemic or contact with infected people.

2. Blood Tests: Blood is drawn for laboratory analysis. Enzyme-linked immunosorbent assay (ELISA) and polymerase chain reaction (PCR) assays are specific diagnostic procedures used to look for Marburg virus genetic material or antibodies in blood.

3. Virus Isolation: From the patient's blood or other bodily fluids, an attempt may be undertaken to isolate the live virus. Due to the virus's high level of contagiousness, this is frequently done in high-containment labs.

4. Differential diagnosis: Before confirming an MVD diagnosis, medical professionals must rule out other possible causes because the early symptoms of MVD can match those of other infectious diseases including malaria, typhoid fever, or Ebola.

5. Imaging: To determine the extent of organ involvement, chest X-rays or computed tomography (CT) scans may be utilized, particularly if the patient comes with significant respiratory symptoms or pulmonary edema.

6. Contact tracing: In the event of an outbreak, locating and keeping track of

people who may have been exposed to the virus is crucial. These people are closely watched for any indications of sickness.

A prompt and correct MVD diagnosis is essential for managing patients, isolating them, and containing outbreaks. Healthcare professionals and laboratory staff handling samples suspected of having Marburg virus must adhere to strict biosafety standards to prevent inadvertent exposure and additional virus dissemination due to the risk of transmission and the severity of the disease.

Is there a treatment for MVD?

The Marburg virus disease (MVD) is not specifically treated with an antiviral medication. However, supportive care is essential in the management of the illness, and a number of treatments can increase a patient's chances of recovery:

1. Intravenous fluids: Due to symptoms including vomiting and diarrhea, patients with MVD frequently get dehydrated. Fluids administered intravenously (IV) support electrolyte balance and hydration.

2. Pain and Fever Management: Acetaminophen and similar drugs can be used to treat pain and lower fever. Due to the possibility of bleeding, non-steroidal anti-inflammatory medicines (NSAIDs) are typically avoided.

3. Blood Transfusions: Severe MVD cases may cause bleeding and coagulation problems. To treat bleeding issues, blood transfusions with clotting components or platelets may be required.

4. Oxygen Therapy: If a patient experiences respiratory distress, more oxygen may be given to help them breathe.

5. Treatment of Complications: Patients with MVD may experience particular interventions such as organ failure. For instance, dialysis may be required if you have kidney failure.

6. Isolation: Strict isolation protocols are essential to stop the virus from spreading to other patients and healthcare personnel.

Antiviral medicines and monoclonal antibodies are examples of experimental treatments and therapies that have been investigated in preclinical trials and occasionally used compassionately during outbreaks. The effectiveness and safety of these treatments haven't been proven beyond a doubt, though.

Is there a vaccine for MVD?

The MVD caused by the Marburg virus has no approved vaccination. However, there has been ongoing research and development into the creation of vaccines for MVD and related filoviruses like Ebola.

To evaluate the safety and effectiveness of different vaccination candidates, including experimental vaccines, preclinical and clinical trials were being conducted. These vaccinations sought to elicit an immunological reaction against the Marburg virus and perhaps offer defense against the illness.

A number of vaccination platforms, including protein subunit vaccines and viral vectors (such as vaccines based on the vesicular stomatitis virus), were being researched. Early-stage clinical studies of some experimental vaccines revealed encouraging outcomes, and their development proceeded.

What are the prevention measures for MVD?

To reduce the risk of exposure and transmission, strict precautions must be taken in the prevention of Marburg virus disease (MVD). Important preventive steps include:

1. Avoiding Contact with Those Who Are Infected: Keep a safe distance away from people who have been identified as having MVD. Keep infected people apart to avoid coming into contact with their bodily fluids.

2. Hand Hygiene: Wash your hands frequently and thoroughly with soap and water or use hand sanitizers with at least 60% alcohol, particularly after coming into touch with objects or people that could be contaminated.

3. Personal Protective Equipment (PPE): To prevent contact with infectious bodily fluids, healthcare professionals and others who come into close contact with MVD patients should wear the proper PPE, such as gloves, masks, gowns, and eye protection.

4. Safe Burial Practices: When dealing with people who have died from MVD, use safe burial procedures. Wearing safety equipment

and avoiding customary funeral rites that require intimate contact with the dead are part of this.

5. Infection Control: To prevent nosocomial (hospital-acquired) infections, healthcare facilities should follow stringent infection control protocols that include isolating suspected patients, following strict hygiene procedures, and sterilizing medical equipment.

6. Community Education: Spread knowledge about the virus, its transmission, and protective measures in populations at risk for MVD. Encourage people to immediately report any suspicious cases.

7. Animal Contact: Steer clear of wildlife such as bats and non-human primates that can act as Marburg virus reservoirs. To reduce the danger of zoonotic transmission, use proper food preparation and cooking techniques.

8. Travelers should take care to prevent contact with potentially infected animals and people in areas where the Marburg virus is endemic. Follow local health advice and guidelines.

9. Support continuing research and surveillance projects to track the existence of the Marburg virus in animal and human

populations, enabling early discovery and outbreak response.

10. Vaccination (when accessible): If a risk-free and efficient vaccine becomes available, think about getting one. Keep up with new advancements in vaccines and advice from medical professionals.

Due to its high death rate and propensity for rapid spread within hospital environments and communities, MVD prevention is crucial. These preventative measures can help lower the danger of exposure and safeguard both individual health and the general public's health.

CHAPTER 2: THE MARBURG VIRUS: A CLOSER LOOK

As a powerful and deadly pathogen, the Marburg virus, a member of the Filoviridae family, claims our attention. This microscopic organism was first identified in 1967 after an outbreak in Marburg, Germany, and has since drawn significant scientific attention and widespread concern.

The Marburg virus is distinguished by its filamentous and frequently twisted form, which it shares with its infamous cousin, the Ebola virus. Both cause hemorrhagic fevers with significant fatality rates, with Marburg virus disease (MVD) developing a reputation as a cunning and evasive adversary.

MVD has historically flourished in situations where human interaction with sick species, such as bats and primates, is frequent. It is spread through direct contact with the blood, saliva, or other bodily fluids of infected individuals. Due to this mechanism of transmission and the severity of its contagiousness, MVD poses a serious risk to the public's health.

A battery of diagnostic investigations, including blood analysis and attempts at virus isolation, are essential to the diagnosis of MVD. We continue to search for a specific antiviral therapy for MVD, but to no avail. The mainstay of treatment is supportive care, which includes blood transfusions, pain control, and hydration.

Thus, the best line of protection against this deadly foe is prevention. Strict measures include avoiding contact with infected people, maintaining effective infection control in hospital settings, sticking to safe burial procedures, and exercising thorough hand cleanliness.

Researchers keep looking into new vaccines and treatments in the pursuit of a more optimistic future. The Marburg virus serves as a stark reminder of the necessity of improving our knowledge, readiness, and awareness to tackle new infectious diseases on a worldwide scale. Its complex molecular makeup and catastrophic effects.

The virus itself

The Marburg virus's distinctive traits, which contribute to its renown and virulence, are present in the virus itself. It stands out visually because of its filamentous structure, which frequently exhibits exquisite twists and turns. This tiny thing is enclosed in genetic material that contains the instructions for its destructive consequences.

The virus enters the host's cells directly by direct contact with infected bodily fluids and then uses the host's cells as its own to proliferate ruthlessly. Its genetic code controls the creation of viral proteins, which disturbs regular cellular processes.

The Marburg virus actively attacks the host's immune system as it replicates while evading identification and treatment. The virus's capacity to avoid immune responses aids in its quick transmission and unrestrained proliferative growth inside the body.

This viral invasion has significant clinical repercussions. A series of symptoms, such as a fever, chills, muscle discomfort, and crippling weakness, are brought on by it. The host is further weakened by gastrointestinal symptoms such nausea, vomiting, and diarrhea. In severe situations, the virus causes organ failure and hemorrhagic complications, sealing the terrible fate of its victim.

The Marburg virus continues to be a powerful foe despite the scientific community's diligent efforts. The lack of a specialized antiviral therapy leaves healthcare practitioners with few options and forces them to rely extensively on supportive care techniques to lessen the effects.

Continuous study and attentive surveillance are crucial as we deal with the problems this virus has brought forth. The secret to unlocking the virus's secrets and creating powerful countermeasures to its destructive impacts on both individual health and global public wellbeing lies in a closer look at the virus itself.

How the virus spreads

The virus uses its ability to penetrate and spread within host organisms to spread through a variety of complex methods. Direct contact with bodily fluids that are infected is the main method of transmission, acting as a conduit for the disease's sneaky spread.

1. Human-to-Human Transmission: Through close, unprotected contact, the virus can spread from one person to another. This includes coming into contact with an infected

person's blood, saliva, vomit, urine, feces, and other bodily secretions. The risk of transmission is considerably increased when a person is physically close to an infected individual, particularly in healthcare environments or when providing care.

2. Inadequate Infection Control Measures and Contaminated Medical Equipment: In healthcare facilities, both of these factors might contribute to the spread of the virus. Instruments that have not been properly sterilized or disinfected can act as transmission vectors.

3. Burial Procedures: Transmission can occur as a result of improper burial procedures that

involve intimate touch with the deceased, who may still be carrying the virus. Individuals may be put at risk by traditional practices that entail cleaning, touching, or handling the body.

4. Zoonotic Transmission: Although less often, the virus can spread from animals to people. The Marburg virus is known to exist naturally in bats in particular. The virus can spread to human populations through close contact with infected wildlife or through the ingestion of contaminated animals.

5. Nosocomial Transmission: If correct infection control procedures are not strictly adhered to within healthcare institutions, the

virus can result in nosocomial (hospital-acquired) infections. Healthcare professionals are more at risk if they come into contact with infected patients or their bodily fluids.

6. Community Outbreaks: The Marburg virus can quickly spread within communities in areas where it is endemic or during outbreaks. Close-knit social networks and events can be a source of transmission since there, people may unintentionally come into touch with infected persons.

In order to adopt efficient preventative measures, break the chain of infection, and control Marburg virus outbreaks, it is crucial to comprehend these ways of transmission. To slow the spread of the virus, vigilance, strict infection control, and public health awareness are essential.

How the virus affects the body

The virus enters the body with ruthless precision, setting off a chain of events that severely impairs regular physiological processes. How the virus impacts the body is as follows:

1. Viral Invasion: The virus targets particular cells as soon as it enters the body, frequently immune cells and endothelial cells lining blood arteries. Through attaching to cell

surface receptors, it infiltrates cells and takes control of their machinery.

2. Replication: Once a virus has entered a host cell, it uses the cellular machinery to duplicate its genetic material and create viral proteins. Within the host, a rising army of viral particles is produced by this quick replication process.

3. Immune Evasion: To get past the immune system's defenses, the virus employs a number of different techniques. It can alter immunological responses and decrease the host's ability to produce interferons, which are necessary antiviral proteins, making it

more challenging for the immune system to recognize and successfully treat the infection.

4. Systemic Inflammation: A strong inflammatory response brought on by the viral invasion results in the release of pro-inflammatory cytokines. The intensity of symptoms may be increased by the broad inflammation that this "cytokine storm" may cause throughout the body.

5. When Symptoms Start: As the virus spreads and multiplies, it causes a variety of symptoms. These frequently include weariness, headaches, muscle soreness, chills, and fever. These earliest signs of infection serve as a warning.

6. Gastrointestinal Distress: Some virus-infected people endure stomach pain, nausea, vomiting, and diarrhea, which further deteriorates the host's health.

Hemorrhagic consequences can result from a virus that, in severe situations, interferes with the blood-clotting cascade. This may cause easy bruising, bleeding gums and nose, bloody vomit, bloody diarrhea, and all of the above.

8. Multi-Organ Failure: The virus may induce multi-organ failure as it continues to attack the body. Organs like the liver, kidneys, and

lungs may develop malfunction, which compromises essential body processes.

9. Respiratory Distress: The infected person may experience severe respiratory symptoms, such as pulmonary edema and acute respiratory distress syndrome (ARDS), which make breathing more challenging.

10. Shock and Death: In the most severe cases, the virus-induced shock and organ failure can be lethal, resulting in a quick demise.

The virus's horrifying effects on the body highlight how urgently we need to do research to develop cures and vaccines. For successful interventions to reduce the impacts of infection and stop the transmission of the virus, it is essential to comprehend these effects.

CHAPTER 3: MARBURG VIRUS DISEASE: CASE STUDIES

Real-world Marburg virus disease (MVD) cases can be examined to gain important knowledge about the disease's clinical development, modes of transmission, and public health responses. Case studies of note are as follows:

1. The Index Case, which occurred in 1967 in Marburg, Germany:

The first known instance of Marburg Virus Disease (MVD) was discovered in 1967 in the German city of Marburg. Workers in a lab processing imported African green monkeys unintentionally handled infected tissues and blood samples. Several employees

47

subsequently experienced serious symptoms, including organ failure, a high fever, and bleeding tendencies. Measures for seclusion and prompt medical assistance were put in place. The Marburg virus was discovered as a result of this important case, which also signaled the start of MVD research.

2. The MVD Epidemic in Uganda in 2007: Uganda experienced a severe MVD outbreak in 2007. After visiting a cave with diseased bats, a family in the Luwero District became ill. The infection swiftly spread across the family, killing off several people. Through stringent isolation procedures, detailed contact tracking, and community awareness campaigns, the outbreak was successfully

limited, highlighting the crucial role that public health interventions play in stopping transmission.

3. The 2012 MVD Outbreak in Uganda: The Kibaale District was the site of the 2012 MVD Outbreak in Uganda. A healthcare professional who had cared for a patient with MVD unintentionally contracted the disease. This example stressed the vital necessity for strict infection control measures within healthcare facilities and brought attention to the increased susceptibility of healthcare workers.

4. The Koltsovo Outbreak, 2004: In the Russian city of Koltsovo in 2004, there was

an MVD outbreak. This outbreak was linked to a lab accident in which a scientist unintentionally came into contact with the Marburg virus. Further transmission was averted by prompt identification of the exposure and prompt application of stringent isolation and treatment measures. The incident made clear how crucially important strict biosafety procedures are in high-containment laboratories.

5. The Durba Outbreak, 1998–2000 :

A protracted MVD outbreak took place in Durban, Democratic Republic of the Congo, between 1998 and 2000. Workers in gold mines who came into contact with diseased bats up close were blamed for the outbreak.

Within the mining community, the virus spread quickly, resulting in a sizable number of cases. Case isolation, contact tracing, and community education about preventive measures were all part of the containment efforts.

6. The Angola Epidemic of 2005: The first known MVD outbreak in Angola occurred in 2005. There were many cases because the virus spread in close-knit communities and medical facilities. The outbreak sparked a global response, highlighting the value of international cooperation in controlling and reducing MVD outbreaks.

These case studies shed light on the many environments in which MVD has arisen and the various difficulties that healthcare systems and communities have encountered in containing it. They act as somber reminders of the continual requirement for awareness, readiness, and research to combat this powerful infectious disease.

CHAPTER 4: THE FUTURE OF MARBURG VIRUS DISEASE

The future of Marburg virus disease (MVD) is at a turning point, with several crucial developments and factors to be taken into account:

1. Vaccine research: Ongoing initiatives in this area provide encouragement for MVD prevention. Preclinical and clinical testing on promising candidates has increased the likelihood of developing a potent MVD vaccine that can prevent outbreaks and protect populations at risk.

2. Antiviral Therapies: Research into particular antiviral medications is ongoing with the goal of creating Marburg virus-specific medicines. Patients may have options with these treatments, especially in the absence of a vaccination.

3. Worldwide Surveillance and Preparedness: For early identification and response to MVD epidemics, improved worldwide surveillance systems are essential. To stop the virus's quick spread, public health infrastructures must be built and strengthened both in endemic areas and globally.

4. Community Involvement and Education: Community awareness and involvement are

essential to the prevention of MVD. Communities can be made more resilient by educating members of the population about the virus, how it spreads, and how to take precautions.

5. Healthcare Worker Training: It is still crucial to train healthcare staff on biosafety procedures and infection control. Providing them with the information and resources they need to safely manage MVD cases is crucial for lowering transmission that is connected to healthcare.

6. Continued investigation into the biology, epidemiology, and host interactions of the virus is crucial. The development of effective

MVD therapies, diagnostics, and vaccinations will be fueled by technological advances.

7. International Cooperation: It is essential for governments, researchers, healthcare facilities, and humanitarian organizations to collaborate internationally. A cohesive response to MVD epidemics is made possible through coordinated actions, which lessens the virus's effects.

8. One Health Approach: Given the zoonotic nature of the Marburg virus, it is crucial to use a "One Health" approach that takes into account the interdependence of human, animal, and environmental health. For

spillover occurrences to be avoided, it is essential to track and comprehend the virus' existence in wildlife reservoirs.

Our shared dedication to research, readiness, and response will determine how the Marburg virus disease develops in the future. There is optimism that the severe effects of MVD can be reduced, assuring a safer and healthier future for everybody, as scientific development and international cooperation continue to advance.

What are the challenges of preventing and treating MVD?

Due to the traits of the virus and the various circumstances in which it can originate, treating and preventing Marburg virus disease (MVD) presents a number of severe problems. These are the main difficulties:

1. Lack of Licensed Vaccines: The lack of Licensed MVD Vaccines is one of the main problems. It takes a lot of time and money to develop and test vaccines for a rare and sporadic illness like Marburg.

2. Limited Treatment Options: MVD is not currently being treated with any specific antiviral medications. Extensive investigation and meticulous clinical testing are required for the development of effective medications.

3. High Contagiousness: MVD is extremely communicable, particularly in medical settings. Strict infection control procedures and protective gear are necessary to stop transmission, however these items may be hard to come by in locations with a lack of resources.

4. Changing Transmission Dynamics: During an outbreak, the virus's transmission dynamics might alter, making containment difficult. It takes flexibility and resources to recognize and react to novel transmission patterns.

5. Community Involvement: Community involvement in impacted areas is essential for

prevention. The distrust of healthcare systems and strongly rooted cultural traditions, however, might obstruct community mobilization and education initiatives.

6. Wildlife Reservoirs: It is challenging to monitor and manage the Marburg virus's natural reservoirs, such as bats. A never-ending issue is preventing incidents where animals affect humans.

7. Surveillance Gaps: In areas with limited resources, MVD surveillance frequently experiences gaps, making it difficult to quickly identify and contain epidemics.

8. Healthcare Worker Risk: Because of their frequent interaction with MVD patients, healthcare workers are at a significant risk of contracting an infection. In environments with limited resources, it is crucial but frequently difficult to ensure their safety through training and appropriate protective gear.

9. Outbreak Response: Delayed reactions might allow the virus to spread more widely and rapid deployment of resources and expertise to outbreak locations can be logistically challenging.

10. Research Obstacles: Scientists face logistical and safety difficulties since

studying MVD involves access to the virus and high-containment labs.

11. Limited Public Awareness: It might be challenging to alter behaviors and practices when people are not aware of MVD and its dynamics of transmission.

Governments, global organizations, scholars, and neighborhood groups must work together in a multidisciplinary manner to address these issues. Additionally, it calls for continued investment and dedication to increase research, monitoring, and Marburg virus disease readiness.

What are the prospects for a vaccine?

With significant advancements in vaccine production and ongoing research efforts, the chances for a vaccine against the Marburg virus disease (MVD) are looking promising. The positive outlook is influenced by a number of factors:

1. Vaccine Candidates: Several potential vaccines have been created and are presently undergoing preclinical and clinical testing. These contenders use a range of tools, such as viral vectors, protein subunits, and other cutting-edge techniques.

2. Positive Results: Early-stage clinical trials and animal research have shown efficacy and

safety of some investigational vaccines for MVD. These successful results lay a solid platform for future growth.

3. Cross-Protection with Ebola: Because Marburg and Ebola viruses share a close genetic link, some vaccine candidates may offer cross-protection, which is advantageous in areas where both viruses may coexist.

4. International Collaboration: Governments, academic institutions, and pharmaceutical corporations working together internationally to further research and development initiatives. Collaboration-based projects speed up vaccine development and enable resource sharing.

5. Funding Commitment: Governments and global health organizations have committed significant funding and assistance to the development of vaccines against filoviruses, particularly Marburg virus.

6. Lessons from Ebola: The effective creation and use of Ebola vaccines during recent outbreaks have taught important lessons and offered a framework for the creation of MVD vaccines.

While there has been progress, there are still obstacles to overcome, such as the requirement for extensive clinical trials to evaluate vaccination safety and effectiveness across a range of groups. Additionally, logistical difficulties for vaccine development and dissemination may arise because of the rarity of MVD and the scarcity of resources in affected areas.

To develop a successful MVD vaccine, more research, cooperation, and financing are required. In order to avoid and lessen the effects of Marburg virus disease epidemics, the global health community is still committed to improving this crucial area of research.

CHAPTER 5: MARBURG VIRUS DISEASE: WHAT YOU CAN DO

Individuals, communities, and healthcare professionals can take proactive measures to protect themselves and support prevention efforts in the face of Marburg virus disease (MVD). What you can do is:

1. Maintain Good Hand Hygiene: Wash your hands frequently for at least 20 seconds with soap and water. Use hand sanitizer with at least 60% alcohol if soap and water are not available.

2. Practice respiratory hygiene. When you cough or sneeze, cover your mouth and nose

with a tissue or your elbow. Use proper disposal for used tissues.

3. Avoid Close Contact: Keep a safe distance from those who are showing signs of MVD and heed public health advice on keeping a social distance while an outbreak is present.

4. Use Personal Protective Equipment (PPE): When caring for patients with MVD, healthcare staff should follow stringent infection control procedures and use the proper PPE.

5. Safe Burial Practices: If you participate in burial customs, abide by safe burial rules to avoid transmission from the dead.

6. Stay Informed: Keep current with news about MVD epidemics, preventative strategies, and travel advice from credible health organizations and governmental organizations.

7. Community Awareness: Take part in community awareness campaigns to inform others about MVD, how it spreads, and how to take precautions. Encourage people to immediately report any suspicious cases.

Supporting research and monitoring initiatives is essential for keeping track of the Marburg virus's existence in both animal and human populations. Promote the provision of financing and resources to support these efforts.

9. Vaccination (when available): If an effective and safe MVD vaccine becomes available, you should think about getting it, especially if you reside in or frequently visit at-risk areas.

10. Be Prepared: Be ready with necessary equipment and knowledge about how to protect yourself and your family in areas where MVD is endemic or during outbreaks.

11. Healthcare Workers: To safely handle MVD cases, make sure you have received

training in infection control and biosafety procedures if you work in healthcare.

12. Report Symptoms: If you or someone you know begins to have symptoms that are consistent with MVD, get help right once and let your doctor know about any possible exposure history.

It is essential to take both group and individual responsibility in order to stop the spread of the Marburg virus sickness. We may contribute to preserving the general public's health and lessening the effects of MVD epidemics by following these recommendations and maintaining our knowledge.

What can communities and governments do to prevent and respond to MVD outbreaks?

Communities and governments are essential in both preventing and controlling epidemics of the Marburg virus disease (MVD). What they can do is:

Communities:

1. Raising awareness and educating people: Communities can inform their citizens about MVD, how it spreads, and how to take precautions. This includes distributing information via local media, schools, and community leaders.

2. Promote safe burial techniques that reduce the chance of transmission during funeral ceremonies. Encourage good hygiene habits including consistent handwashing and proper respiratory care.

3. Encourage people to notify local health officials as soon as they suspect a case of MVD. Timely response depends on early discovery.

4. Support efforts to isolate and confine infected people as well as those who have been exposed to the virus. Communities can help those who are impacted by providing services and assistance.

5. Contact Tracing: Help health authorities identify people who may have been exposed to the virus by supporting contact tracing activities.

6. Community Health Workers: Prepare and train community health workers to offer fundamental medical care, keep an eye out for symptoms, and inform the local population about MVD.

Governments:

1. Surveillance and Reporting: Develop effective surveillance programs to track possible MVD cases and atypical illness

trends. Make sure medical facilities promptly report suspicious instances.

2. Emergency Response Plans: For MVD outbreaks, create and often update detailed emergency response plans. Protocols for isolation, treatment, and contact tracing should be included in these preparations.

3. Resource Allocation: Distribute resources, such as money, people, and medical equipment, to respond to outbreaks successfully. Make sure that medical facilities have enough space and safety gear.

Launch public health campaigns to inform the populace about MVD, preventive actions, and the need of early reporting.

5. International Collaboration: Exchange knowledge, resources, and skills with international health organizations and surrounding nations. Because MVD outbreaks can spread across borders, a coordinated response is required.

6. Vaccination Programs: When reliable vaccines are developed, support the development and execution of MVD vaccination programs. Give vaccinations for at-risk groups and healthcare personnel top priority.

7. Community Involvement: Work to foster cooperation in epidemic response initiatives by interacting with regional communities.

8. Research and Development: Invest in this field to create therapies, enhance diagnostic equipment, and gain a better understanding of the virus.

Communities and governments must work together in a concerted effort to prevent MVD epidemics and respond to them. They can lessen the effects of MVD on public health and stop its spread by proactively addressing the virus's threat and putting in place thorough procedures.

Conclusion

In conclusion, Marburg virus disease (MVD) continues to be a dangerous infectious disease with a wide range of obstacles. MVD is a strong foe due to the lack of approved vaccinations, specialized antiviral medications, and the virus's high contagiousness. Communities, governments, medical professionals, and researchers all have important roles to play in stopping and controlling MVD outbreaks.

With continuous research and vaccine development efforts yielding promising outcomes, the future of MVD is bright. However, combating this disease's problems calls for ongoing commitment, funding, and international cooperation.

We can lower the likelihood of MVD transmission and lessen its effects on people and communities by increasing public awareness, educating the public, promoting early detection, and implementing strict infection control measures. There is hope for a future in which MVD is a treatable and preventable disease thanks to the knowledge gained from previous outbreaks and the dedication of people and organizations around the world.

Our collaborative efforts to comprehend, stop, and treat Marburg virus sickness in the face of this powerful pathogen serve as a ray of hope and fortitude in the field of infectious diseases.